ESSENTIAL HERBS:

BENEFITS & USES OF GINGER, RECIPES WITH GINGER

JOSEPH VEEBE

Books in this Series:

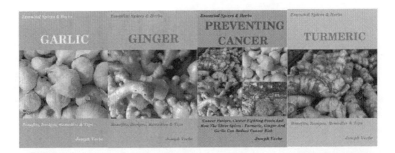

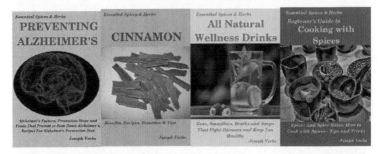

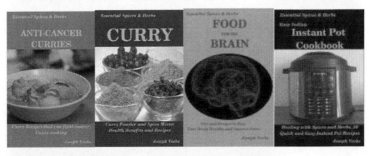

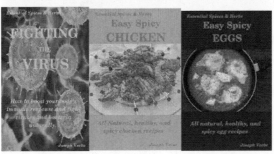

TABLE OF CONTENTS

Chapter 1. Introduction and history

Introduction

I want to thank you for purchasing this book, "Essential Spices & Herbs: Ginger." This is the second book in the "Essential Spices and Herbs" series. This book lists the health benefits of ginger, a spice known to man for thousands of years. Recent studies have shown that ginger has many properties including anticancer, antioxidant, and anti-inflammatory properties. The book also details how to incorporate ginger in your daily diet. Several easy to use recipes are described that I hope the reader finds useful.

There are several spices and herbs used by ancient civilizations with proven and time-tested health benefits. Modern medicine has been increasingly studying many of these herbs and spices. However, more organized studies that are needed to get approval from the regulatory agencies for these herbs and spices to be accepted as part of mainstream prevention or treatment options for some medical conditions.

In this day and age of 'superfoods,' organic foods, healthy cooking, and eating, one of the often-neglected areas is the use of spices and herbs in cooking and diet plans.

We all want to eat healthy and tasty food. But we are all too busy to make fresh food at home. So, we settle for fast foods or packaged foods instead of healthy, fresh foods. The recipes listed in this book are quick and easy. The average time to make the recipes is about 20 minutes.

Many of us have heard that spices and herbs are good for health, but we hardly incorporate these in western cuisine. Even though there is more awareness lately on the health benefits of herbs/spices as part of the natural alternative to medicines, only a very few that regularly incorporate spices and herbs in their diet. Some people hit nutritional stores to get natural supplements. While supplements are in general good, getting the same through natural foods is preferable.

The recipes in the book are put together so that they can be easily prepared using ingredients that are commonly available. There are several optional ingredients that you can try out to make the dish according to your taste and creativity. The book will also cover uses beyond dietary and cooking using these spices.

HISTORY

Humans have used spices since the beginning of time. One can find references to various spices in ancient scripts such as the Old Testament, Bhagavad-Gita, and other writings. Ancient Egyptians, Chinese, Indians, Arabs, Greece, and Rome have all used spices for various purposes, from cooking to food preservation and as medicine. Many things attracted humans to the use of spices – their aroma, the distinct taste and its ability to flavor food, their color, and last but not least their medicinal properties. Spices also helped early humans to preserve food and other things. Archeologists discovered the use of spices in ancient Egyptian tombs and other excavations. There are records of many civilizations around the world using herbs and spices for common ailments such as wound healing, fever, and microbial infections.

GINGER – THE TONIC ROOT

Ginger (*Zingiber officinale*) is a flowering plant whose root is widely used as a spice and traditional medicine over thousands of years in Asia. Ginger belongs to the same family as turmeric and cardamom.

Ginger is widely used in Asian cooking, especially China and India. While turmeric, which belongs to the same family as ginger is mostly used in the powder form, ginger is used as a fresh ingredient in most cooking. This book will focus on ginger and its benefits as part of food and cooking.

Ginger is one of the key ingredients in Asian cuisine for years. Ginger is a necessary ingredient in almost all of the meat recipes in Indian cooking. Ginger, when dried and ground results in a white powder that is used in baking (gingerbread, cookies, crackers, cakes, etc.) and also making beverages (ginger ale, ginger beer, etc.). Ginger, either powdered or fresh, can be used in teas and is an essential component of 'masala chai'.

The main bioactive active ingredient in ginger is called gingerol and it has very powerful medicinal properties. Ginger is used in several alternative/traditional medicines in the East.

CHAPTER 2. NUTRITIONAL INFORMATION

Ginger, unlike turmeric, is not a significant source of vitamins and minerals. More than 75% of raw ginger is water. Ginger does contain small amounts of minerals and vitamins as in the table below. The most important component of ginger is gingerol which provides its anti-oxidant and anti-inflammatory characteristics.

Nutrient data for Ginger root, raw (source USDA)

Nutrient	1 tsp = 2.0g	0.25 cup slices (1" dia) = 24.0g	5.0 slices (1" dia) = 11.0g
Proximates			
Water	1.58g	18.93g	8.68
Energy	2kcal	19kcal	9
Protein	40mg	440mg	0.2
Total lipid (fat)	10mg	180mg	0.08
Carbohydrate, by difference	360mg	4.26g	1.95
Fiber, total dietary	40mg	500mg	200mg
Sugars, total	30mg	410mg	190mg
Minerals			
Calcium, Ca	0.4mg	4mg	2mg
Iron, Fe	10ug	140ug	70ug
Magnesium, Mg	1mg	10mg	5mg
Phosphorus, P	1mg	8mg	4mg
Potassium, K	8mg	100mg	46mg
Sodium, Na	0.2mg	3mg	1mg
Zinc, Zn	10ug	80ug	40ug
Vitamins			
Vitamin C, total ascorbic acid	100ug	1.2mg	600ug
Thiamin	0.6ug	6ug	3ug
Riboflavin	1ug	8ug	4ug
Niacin	15ug	180ug	83ug
Vitamin B-6	3ug	38ug	18ug
Folate, DFE	0.2ug	3ug	1ug
Vitamin B-12	0	0	0

Vitamin A, RAE	0	0	0
Vitamin A, IU	0	0	0
Vitamin E (alpha-tocopherol)	10ug	60ug	30ug
Vitamin D (D2 + D3)	0	0	0
Vitamin D	0	0	0
Vitamin K (phylloquinone)	0	0	0
Lipids			
Fatty acids, total saturated	4mg	49mg	22ug
Fatty acids, total monounsaturated	3mg	37mg	17ug
Fatty acids, total polyunsaturated	3mg	37mg	17ug
Fatty acids, total trans	0	0	0
Cholesterol	0	0	0
Other			
Caffeine	0	0	0

CHAPTER 3. BENEFITS OF GINGER

Ginger has several health benefits. The ginger root, when consumed regularly helps improve the digestive system, when. Ginger is known to reduce the feeling of nausea, and also improve your body's immune system to help fight common ailments such as flu, common cold, fever, etc.

Ginger is available in many different forms – fresh ginger, dried ginger, ginger paste, ginger powder, and ginger supplements. Fresh ginger and ginger paste is used mostly cooking. Dried ginger and ginger powder usually used in baking.

INDIGESTION

Ginger has been used in traditional medicine as a digestive aid for thousands of years. In the East, ginger is an essential ingredient in meat cooking not only to add flavor to the food but also to help in digestion as well. Chewing on fresh ginger or drinking ginger juice/drink can help cure minor tummy aches (due to indigestion) and help with bloating and constipation.

Ginger relieves and relaxes gastrointestinal muscles that help reduce stomach irritation. It also helps in bile production and movement of food through the gastrointestinal tract and thereby helping proper metabolism and food absorption in the body.

NAUSEA AND MORNING SICKNESS

Ginger has been used as a home remedy for different forms of nausea from morning sickness and motion sickness to even nausea due to chemotherapy.

Ginger has been used for motion sickness (seasickness primarily) for centuries. Recent studies have shown that ginger is effective in preventing morning sickness, pregnancy-related nausea.

PAIN

Ginger is considered to help with pain – especially exercise-induced muscle pain. Drinking some ginger juice/drink after exercise regularly may be useful to relieve muscle pain. Also, ginger has been studied for its effectiveness for menstrual pain and cramps and has been found as effective as some of the pain medications.

ANTI-INFLAMMATORY

Ginger has been used for centuries as an anti-inflammatory herb. Recent studies have shown that a steady intake of ginger for a month helped reduce inflammation in the colon. By reducing inflammation, the risk of colon cancer is also reduced. Another study has shown promise in reducing inflammation associated with osteoarthritis.

ANTI-CANCER PROPERTIES

There have been studies conducted on the effects of ginger in colorectal cancer patients that have shown the effectiveness of ginger in arresting the growth of cancer cells. This may not be surprising given how good ginger for the gastrointestinal system. Ginger is believed to be also effective in other forms of cancer such as pancreatic cancer, ovarian cancer, and breast cancer. Further studies are required to confirm these.

IMMUNE SYSTEM & INFECTIONS

As ginger has antioxidant, anti-inflammatory, and anti-microbial properties, its use helps in the improved immune system. Studies have shown that ginger extract can prevent growth or even kill some of the bacteria and viruses. Studies have been conducted on the effects of gingerol against bacteria that cause gingivitis and periodontitis that have shown ginger to be effective against these. Another study has shown that fresh ginger is effective against respiratory infections. Studies have shown that ginger is also effective against fungal infections.

DIABETES AND HEART HEALTH

Ginger is believed to have several properties that help in maintaining a healthy heart including blood thinning, stimulating circulation, reducing cholesterol levels, and preventing heart attacks and strokes.

A study conducted on gingerol effect on blood sugar found that there were significant benefits of using the ginger powder in lowering blood sugar levels in diabetic patients.

CHOLESTEROL

Studies have shown that a daily intake of ginger help reduces LDL cholesterol (bad cholesterol). The studies were conducted in humans as well as animals. As a result, the daily use of ginger may help maintain not only a healthy gut but a healthy heart as well.

NEUROPROTECTIVE

Inflammation and oxidative damage to brain cells is considered the key contributing factors to the accelerated aging process. By consuming anti-oxidant and anti-inflammatory foods, one can reduce the effect of aging on the brain.

Ginger has antioxidant and anti-inflammatory properties that can help with slowing down the age-related decline in brain function such as Alzheimer's diseases.

CHAPTER 4. RECIPES WITH GINGER

There are several ways to incorporate ginger into your everyday diet. Some basic ideas are:

- Add a small piece of ginger root in the blender while making smoothies
- Add ginger powder in while baking
- Add ginger paste (or ginger-garlic paste) to a make marinade for grilling meat or fish
- Add a piece of fresh ginger while making tea.
- Juice a piece of ginger and use the ginger juice in teas, cooking.

DRINKS

Ginger may be used to make drinks such as 'masala chai' and smoothies. There are several ways to make ginger tea or masala tea. While Ginger is the main ingredient, adding or mixing and matching other spices and herbs may help create the unique ginger tea or smoothie to your liking.

Most of the recipes below use grated or sliced ginger. Ginger may be pressed to juice and ginger juice may be used to substitute sliced ginger in the recipes below.

BASIC GINGER TEA

Ingredients:

- ½-2 inch fresh ginger, grated
- 1-2 cups of water

Method

1. Add grated ginger to water and boil it for a couple of minutes.
2. Let it cool for a couple of minutes.
3. Filter ginger slices; stir and enjoy warm.

BLACK TEA WITH GINGER AND CARDAMOM

Ingredients:

- ½-1inch fresh ginger, peeled and sliced/crushed
- 1 tsp honey (or as much to sweeten the tea to your taste)
- 1-2 cups of water
- 1 black tea bag
- 2 cardamom pods
- ½ teaspoon lemon juice (optional)

Method

1. Add the ginger slices and optional cardamom to 1-2 cups of water and boil.
2. Add the black tea bag.
3. Let it cool for a couple of minutes.
4. Remove tea bag, filter ginger slices; add honey, and enjoy warm.

You can also try the same by adding optional ½ teaspoon lemon juice.

MASALA CHAI (SPICED TEA)

There are several ways to make masala chai. When I make, I usually use ginger and cardamom only. The other ingredients to add based on one's taste are cinnamon, cloves, and pepper and fennel seeds.

Basic Ingredients

- ½ inch – 1 inch fresh peeled, ginger grated or crushed
- 4-6 cardamoms crushed
- 1 inch long cinnamon stick or ¼ tsp cinnamon powder
- 2-4 tsp brown sugar (optional)
- ½ cup 2% milk
- 3 cups of water
- 2-4 tsp black tea or 2-3 tea bags

Optional Ingredients

- 2-4 cloves
- ¼ tsp pepper powder or about 4 peppercorns
- ¼ teaspoon fennel seeds

Method

1. Grind or crush cardamom, cinnamon, and optional cloves, fennel seeds, and pepper in a spice grinder or mortar.
2. In a pan, add the ground mix and ginger and pour 3 cups of water. Mix it well and bring it to a boil.
3. Reduce heat and let it simmer for a minute or two.

4. Now add the tea, mix, and let it boil for one minute on low heat.
5. Add milk and sugar and mix well. Strain out all the ingredients and enjoy.

If you have not tried masala chai before, I suggest you start with ginger and cardamom and then introduce other items as you like and settle on the ingredient you like best.

GINGER AND LEMON TEA

Ingredients

- ½ inch – 1 inch fresh ginger, grated or crushed
- ½ tsp lemon juice
- 1 tsp honey

Method

1. Boil 2 cups of water in a saucepan.
2. Add ginger and let it boil for 2-3 minutes.
3. Remove from heat and add lemon. Add honey and enjoy warm

Note: This drink is good for nausea. Drink as often as needed. Optionally one can put a black tea bag and make it ginger and lemon black tea. Try various combinations cardamom, cinnamon, and lemon along with ginger with black and settle on the one you like.

Instead of grating, ginger may be pressed to make ginger juice and then combine with lemon juice in hot water and add honey. I had this tea at the Malibu farm café at Malibu Pier in California. They used 2-3 inches of ginger for 1 cup of water and it was very strong and really good.

GINGER ALE

Ingredients

- 1 cup ginger, peeled and sliced or crushed
- 2-3 cups of water
- ½ -1 cup brown sugar
- 1 spoon freshly squeezed lemon juice

Method

1. Add ginger to boiling water and simmer it for 10-15 minutes. Stir well.
2. Add sugar and let it fully dissolve.
3. Put off the heat and let it sit until warm.
4. Strain the ginger pieces. Add lemon juice and stir. Pour the contents into a glass jar and refrigerate it.

The mixture may be used as-is (one spoon at a time) for nausea and indigestion or heartburn. You can also add 4-5 teaspoons of this mixture into a glass of club soda and drink.

TROPICAL SMOOTHIE

Ingredients

- ½ inch – 1 inch fresh ginger, peeled and sliced
- 1 tsp honey (optional to taste)
- 1 banana
- 1 cup pineapple, mango or papaya
- 1 cup of milk or ½ cup plain yogurt.
- ½ cup ice
- ½ inch fresh turmeric (optional)

Method

Process all the ingredients in a blender until smooth.

GREEN SMOOTHIE

Basic Ingredients

- 1 inch fresh ginger, peeled and sliced
- 1 tsp honey (optional to taste)
- 1 cup of kale
- 1 cup spinach
- 1-2 kiwi peeled
- ½ cup blueberries
- 1-2 cup filtered water (coconut water may be used as well)
- ½ cup ice

Optional Ingredients

- ½ cup sliced cucumber, or Italian squash
- ¼ avocado
- 3-4 mint leaves
- ½ inch fresh peeled turmeric root (optional)

Method

Process all the ingredients in a blender until smooth. Blueberry may be substituted by blackberry depending on your liking. Servers 4-5. By mixing and matching "the green" ingredients, you may try a couple of different green smoothies.

GOLDEN YELLOW SMOOTHIE

Ingredients

- 1 inch fresh ginger, grated or thinly sliced (optional)
- 1 tsp honey (optional to taste)
- 1 carrot washed and cut into pieces
- 1 mango peeled and sliced
- 1 cup Orange or Mango Juice
- ½ cup ice

Method

Process all the ingredients in a blender until smooth.

YOGURT WITH TURMERIC, GINGER, AND GARLIC

This is a popular curry in Indian cooking and has several different variations. The simplest version of the recipe is below.

Basic Ingredients

- 1 teaspoon turmeric powder
- ½ inch – 1 inch fresh ginger grated or thinly sliced
- 2-3 cloves of garlic chopped
- 1 pinch of black pepper powder
- 2 cups of yogurt whisked
- 1 medium onion finely chopped
- 2 tsp coconut (or vegetable) oil
- Salt to taste

Optional Ingredients

- ¼ cup cilantro, chopped (optional)
- ¼ cup curry leaves may be used in place of cilantro)
- 1 tsp mustard seeds
- 1 tsp cumin seeds
- 2 crushed red chilies

Method:

1. Heat oil in a medium non-stick pan, add optional mustard seeds, cumin, and red chilies and let it crackle
2. Add onions, ginger, garlic, and optional curry leaves or cilantro.
3. Stir until golden and add turmeric and black pepper, stir for one minute and then add the yogurt and mix well. Switch off the heat and enjoy it with rice.

GINGER, GARLIC AND TURMERIC PASTE

Ginger and garlic paste is used often as part of the marinade in South Asian cooking. Almost all meat recipes use ginger and garlic as ingredients.

The steps below are for making a paste that contains not only ginger and garlic but turmeric as well. This is a powerful combination of ingredients that will not only make your meat tasty but also provide excellent health benefits as well.

Ingredients

- 1 cup ginger washed, peeled and cut into small pieces
- 1 cup garlic – peeled
- ¼ cup turmeric root washed, peeled and cut
- ½ -1 tsp salt
- 1 tsp vegetable oil

Method:

Make sure the ginger and turmeric are dried enough to remove any water from washing. Add all ingredients into a mixer and grind until a smooth paste. Store the contents in a glass jar and use within 3-4 days or a week. The paste may be used as part of any marinade for meat before grilling or baking in the oven or even cooking in a pan.

ENTREES AND OTHER DISHES

BELL PEPPER AND CHICKEN STIR FRY

Ingredients

- 1 bell pepper, washed and cut into thin slices
- 2 tsp coconut oil (olive oil or vegetable oil can be used as well)
- 2 lb. boneless chicken breast cut into 1 inch pieces
- 1 tsp turmeric powder
- 1 tsp black pepper powder
- 1 tsp coriander powder
- 1 medium onion, sliced
- ½ inch piece of ginger, thinly sliced
- Salt to taste
- 1 medium tomato, chopped
- 3 cloves of garlic, chopped
- 1 Jalapeño pepper sliced into thin pieces (optional)
-
- ¼ cup cilantro chopped (optional)

Method

1. Sprinkle ½ spoons of turmeric powder, pepper powder, and salt on the washed and cut chicken, mix well and set aside for 10 minutes.
2. In a pan, heat oil, add onions, crushed garlic, ginger, and optional Jalapeno. Sauté till onions become translucent.
3. Add rest of turmeric powder, coriander powder, and pepper powder and mix well.
4. Add tomato and mix.
5. Now add the bell pepper and chicken and mix well.

6. Cover and cook for 10 minutes on medium heat or until chicken and peppers are cooked. Stir occasionally.
7. Switch off the heat, add optional cilantro, add more salt if required depending on your taste.

Serve with rice or bread

COCONUT CURRY CHICKEN

Basic Ingredients

- 2 lbs. chicken breast, cut into small (1 inch) pieces
- 1-2 tsp of curry powder, depending on your tolerance on spice
- 1 tsp turmeric
- 1` medium onion, chopped
- 2-3 tsp oil
- ½ tsp pepper powder
- 2 medium potatoes – peeled and cut into 1 inch cubes
- 3-4 cloves of garlic crushed
- ½ inch cube of ginger, peeled and chopped
- 1 can (14 oz) of coconut milk
- ¼ cup mint leaves or cilantro
- Salt to taste
- ½ -1 can of chicken broth (depending on the amount gravy desired)

Optional Ingredients

- 1 cup carrot sliced
- 2 medium chopped tomatoes

Method

1. Sprinkle 1 tsp curry powder, ½ turmeric and ¼ tsp salt on cut chicken and mix well and keep it aside for 10 minutes
2. In a separate pan, heat oil, sauté onions, garlic, and ginger until onions become translucent

3. Add remaining curry powder, turmeric and pepper powder, mix for 1-2 minutes,

4. Add chicken and potato and optional tomato and carrot and mix well 1-2 minutes until the chicken and potato are coated with the gravy

5. Add chicken broth and bring it to a boil. Stir well.

6. Reduce heat to low medium, cover the pan and cook for 10-12 minutes or until chicken, potato and carrots are well mixed and chicken loses its pink color and potatoes and carrots are about half cooked.

7. Add coconut milk and cover and simmer on low heat for another 20 minutes or until chicken, potato and carrots are cooked well and soft.

8. Add mint leaves/cilantro and stir. Add salt to taste. Switch off the heat and keep it covered for 1-2 minutes before serving.

Serve with rice or bread.

BEEF/CHICKEN PEPPER FRY

Ingredients

- 2 lbs. boneless chicken breast/beef, cut into 1 inch cubes/stripes
- 2 tsp coconut oil (olive oil or vegetable oil can be used as well)
- 1/2 tsp turmeric powder
- 1-2 tsp black pepper powder
- 2 tsp coriander powder
- 2 large onion sliced
- 2 inch piece of ginger thinly sliced
- Salt to taste
- 2-3 medium tomato sliced
- 4-6 cloves of garlic crushed
- Cilantro – 1 cup (optional)

Method

1. Heat oil in a medium non-stick pan; add onions, garlic, and ginger. Stir until golden
2. Add coriander powder, pepper powder and turmeric, stir for 2-3 minute
3. Add tomato and mix well.
4. Add chicken and mix so that chicken is coated well with spices and onion.
5. Cover and simmer for 20-25 minutes or until the chicken is cooked stirring occasionally so the chicken or the gravy does not stick to the pan.
6. Garnish with cilantro. Serve with rice or naan (Indian bread).

GRILLED CHICKEN

Tandoori chicken is an Indian dish that is marinated in yogurt and spices and cooked in clay oven. It invariably uses a ginger-garlic paste as part of a marinade. Below is a variation of tandoori chicken but made on a grill.

Ingredients

- 2-3 lbs. skinless chicken drumsticks or thighs / alternatively boneless chicken breast cut into pieces.
- 2-3 tsp ginger-garlic paste (see earlier instructions to make it or use store-bought)
- 1 cup low-fat yogurt
- 1 tsp chili powder
- ¼ tsp turmeric powder
- 3 teaspoon tandoori masala (see note below)
- 1 lemon juiced
- 1 cup cilantro (to garnish)
- 2 lemons sliced (to garnish)
- 1 medium onion sliced into long pieces (optional)
- 1 teaspoon salt (or to taste)
- 1 teaspoon oil

Method

The first step is to prepare the marinade.

Marinade Method 1: Mix all the items for the marinade (Yogurt, chili, turmeric, tandoori masala, lemon juice, and ginger garlic paste, salt) into a smooth thick marinade.

Marinade Method 2: Heat oil and fry chili powder, tandoori masala, and turmeric for 2 minutes. Switch the heat and let it cool down. Once cooled, add this to the rest of the ingredients of the marinade and mix well as in the previous step.

1. Put the chicken in a large freezer /ziplock bag and add the marinade. You may want to use multiple freezer bags depending on the quantity but make sure to put sufficient marinade in each bag. Shake the bag well carefully so that the chicken is well coated with the marinade. Refrigerate for a minimum of 2 hrs but preferably 12 hrs. or overnight.

2. When ready to cook, preheat oven to 400 degrees. Take the chicken out of the ziplock bags and carefully place the chicken on a wire rack on the baking dish. The baking dish may be lined with aluminum foil to collect any juice coming out of the chicken. Bake for 25 minutes. Open the oven and apply some oil using a brush on the surface of chicken pieces and turn them over. Bake for another 20 minutes or until cooked well and slightly charred. Take it from the oven. Garnish with cilantro, lemon wedges, and onion slices.

Instead of the oven, the marinated chicken may be barbecued or grilled on an open grill as well.

Note: You can substitute garam masala for tandoori masala. Both of these spice mixes are available in any South Asian store or in the spice section in many grocery stores. You can also make the spice mix by combining the following: 1 tsp coriander powder, 1 tsp pepper powder, 1 tsp cinnamon powder, 1 tsp turmeric powder, ½ tsp cardamom powder (or seeds), 1 tsp chili powder, and ½ tsp nutmeg.

CHAPTER 5. TIPS FOR BUYING AND USING GINGER

COOKING

Ginger has been used in Asian cooking for hundreds of years. Ginger considered an essential ingredient in any meat dish.

Besides flavoring meat and giving it a distinct taste, ginger has been used in folk/traditional medicine for stomach ailments, nausea, common cold, and sore throat. The simplest way to intake ginger is either chewing on a fresh root or making ginger tea or ginger ale.

BUYING

Ginger root is available to buy in both fresh and dried root form as well as in powder form. Almost all grocery stores in North America carry ginger. Ginger paste is usually available in Asian grocery stores. Nutritional and supplement stores carry a wide variety of ginger root extract supplements. Ground ginger or ginger powder is available online and in Asian grocery stores.

GINGER POWDER

While fresh ginger is always preferable, ginger powder is more easily available and has a lot more shelf life, so it is a worthy alternative to fresh ginger. The ginger powder may be added to tea, smoothies, or as part of a spice blend in cooking. Ginger is a perennial plant and may be grown in your own backyard.

GINGER PASTE

Ginger paste is often used as an alternative to fresh ginger and also as part of a marinade for grilling or baking meat. Ginger may be combined with garlic to make ginger garlic paste and stored for several days for use in cooking or marinating meat.

DOSAGE – HOW MUCH GINGER IS APPROPRIATE?

Most of the studies of ginger have used a dosage of 500mg to 2000mg ginger root a day. For children and pregnant women, the dosage is much lower. As always, discuss with your primary care provider before taking any supplements.

GINGER – SOME QUICK HOME REMEDIES

Nausea: Take a warm cup of ginger tea or ginger soda (see ginger drinks section). The same remedy may be used for morning sickness and motion sickness as well.

Cough: grate a piece of ginger and boil it in a cup of water with 2-4 crushed peppercorns. Drink lukewarm with optional honey. The same remedy may be used for a sore throat and flue as well.

Toothache: Chew a piece of ginger for a few days.

Stomach pain/cramps: Drink ginger tea or ginger ale a couple of times a day.

CHAPTER 6. SUMMARY

NUTRITION FACTS

- The active ingredient in ginger is called gingerol

- Gingerol has antioxidant and anti-inflammatory properties among other benefits.

- Contains a substance called 6-gingerol which is believed to be effective against cancer

- A great ingredient for cooking providing unique taste and flavor

GINGER HEALTH BENEFITS

NAUSEA

Effective in many kinds of nausea such as motion sickness, seasickness, morning sickness as well as any other kind

DIGESTIVE SYSTEM

Helps with indigestion, stomach pain and improves the overall health of the digestive system

CANCER

Studies have shown that 6-gingerol, an ingredient in ginger can help prevent prostate and colorectal cancer and has shown cell death in ovarian cancer cells

CHOLESTEROL

According to studies, ginger is beneficial in lowing bad (LDL) cholesterol in your body

GINGER HEALTH BENEFITS

INFECTIONS

Ginger has immune boosting capabilities and can fight common ailments such as cough/cold and flu or fever

PAIN

Ginger can help relieve muscle pain and soreness due to exercise. It is also seen to help joint pain in patients with osteoarthritis

ANTI-INFLAMMATORY

Inflammation is the cause of many diseases and ginger is extremely anti-inflammatory which helps in improved overall health

HEART HEALTH & DIABETES

Studies have shown that ginger can help in improving circulation, thinning the blood and also help with reducing blood sugar

GINGER USAGE

DRINKS

Ginger tea. Smoothies. Ginger Ale. Soups. Add fresh ginger to as part of many drink preparations

COOKING

Cooking meat or vegetables. Pair with Garlic. Use the ginger powder in baking

GINGER PASTE

Prepare ginger paste (or ginger-garlic paste) and keep it for weeks and use it for cooking, preparing a marinade, salad dressing, etc.

GINGER SUPPLEMENTS

Ginger supplements are readily available in nutritional stores and online. Complement supplement as needed along with diet

CHAPTER 7. SOURCES AND REFERENCES

This book was written based on the author's personal experience with the spice as well as information from a wide range of sources. Some of the key sources are outlined below, in case; the reader would like to read more details about ginger and its uses.

Cancer

https://www.ncbi.nlm.nih.gov/pmc/articles/PMC3208778/

http://www.medicalnewstoday.com/articles/150496.php

Pain

https://www.ncbi.nlm.nih.gov/pubmed/19216660

http://www.medicalnewstoday.com/articles/189359.php

Cholesterol

https://www.ncbi.nlm.nih.gov/pubmed/18813412

https://www.ncbi.nlm.nih.gov/pubmed/23901210

Infections

https://www.ncbi.nlm.nih.gov/pubmed/18814211

https://www.ncbi.nlm.nih.gov/pubmed/18814211

https://www.ncbi.nlm.nih.gov/pubmed/23123794

Diabetes & Blood Sugar

https://www.ncbi.nlm.nih.gov/pmc/articles/PMC4277626/

The discovery of spices

http://mccormickscienceinstitute.com/resources/history-of-spices

DISCLAIMER

This book details the author's personal experiences in using Indian spices, the information contained in the public domain as well as the author's opinion. The author is not licensed as a doctor, nutritionist, or chef. The author is providing this book and its contents on an "as is" basis and makes no representations or warranties of any kind with respect to this book or its contents. The author disclaims all such representations and warranties, including for example warranties of merchantability and educational or medical advice for a particular purpose. In addition, the author does not represent or warrant that the information accessible via this book is accurate, complete, or current. The statements made about products and services have not been evaluated by the US FDA or any equivalent organization in other countries.

The author will not be liable for damages arising out of or in connection with the use of this book or the information contained within. This is a comprehensive limitation of liability that applies to all damages of any kind, including (without limitation) compensatory; direct, indirect or consequential damages; loss of data, income or profit; loss of or damage to property and claims of third parties. It is understood that this book is not intended as a substitute for consultation with a licensed medical or a culinary professional. Before starting any lifestyle changes, it is recommended that you consult a licensed professional to ensure that you are doing what's best for your situation. The use of this book implies your acceptance of this disclaimer.

Thank You

If you enjoyed this book or found it useful, I would greatly appreciate if you could post a short review. I read all the reviews and your feedback will help me to make this book even better

PREVIEW OF OTHER BOOKS IN THIS SERIES

ESSENTIAL SPICES AND HERBS: TURMERIC

Turmeric is truly a wonder spice. It has anti-inflammatory, anti-oxidant, anti-cancer, and anti-bacterial properties. Find out the amazing benefits of turmeric. Includes many recipes for incorporating turmeric in your daily life.

Turmeric is a spice known to man for thousands of years and has been used for cooking, food preservation, and as a natural remedy for common ailments. This book explains:

- Many health benefits of turmeric including fighting cancer, inflammation, and pain.
- Turmeric as beauty treatments - turmeric masks
- Recipes for teas, smoothies and dishes
- References and links to a number of research studies on the effectiveness of turmeric

Essential Spices and Herbs: Turmeric is a quick read and offers a lot of concise information. A great tool to have in your alternative therapies and healthy lifestyle toolbox!

PREVENTING CANCER

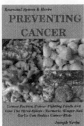 World Health Organization (WHO) estimates more than half of all cancer incidents are preventable.

Cancer is one of the most fearsome diseases to strike mankind. There has been much research into both conventional and alternative therapies for different kinds of cancers. Different cancers require different treatment options and offer a different prognosis. While there has been significant progress in recent times in cancer research towards a cure, there are none available currently. However, more than half of all cancers are likely preventable through modifications in lifestyle and diet.

Preventing Cancer offers a quick insight into cancer-causing factors, foods that fight cancer, and how the three spices, turmeric, ginger and garlic, can not only spice up your food but potentially make all your food into cancer fighting meals. While there are many other herbs and spices that help fight cancer, these three spices work together and complementarily. In addition, the medicinal value of these spices has been proven over thousands of years of use. The book includes:

- Cancer-causing factors and how to avoid them
- Top 12 cancer-fighting foods, the cancers they fight and how to incorporate them into your diet
- Cancer-fighting properties of turmeric, ginger and garlic
- Over 30 recipes including teas, smoothies and other dishes that incorporate these spices

- References and links to many research studies on the effectiveness of these spices.

PREVENTING ALZHEIMER'S

Approximately 50 million people suffer from Alzheimer's worldwide. In the U.S. alone, 5.5 million people have Alzheimer's – about 10 percent of the worldwide Alzheimer's population.

Alzheimer's disease is a progressive brain disorder that damages and eventually destroys brain cells, leading to memory loss, changes in thinking, and other brain functions. While the rate of progressive decline in brain function is slow at the onset, it gets worse with time and age. Brain function decline accelerates, and brain cells eventually die over time. While there has been significant research done to find a cure, currently there is no cure available.

Alzheimer's incidence rate in the U.S. and other western countries is significantly higher than that of the countries in the developing world. Factors such as lifestyle, diet, physical and mental activity, and social engagement play a part in the development and progression of Alzheimer's

In most cases, if you are above the age of 50, plaques and tangles associated with Alzheimer's may have already started forming in your brain. At the age of 65, you have a 10% chance of Alzheimer's and at age 80, the chances are about 50%.

With lifestyle changes, proper diet and exercise (of the mind and body), Alzheimer's is preventable.

In recent times, Alzheimer's is beginning to reach epidemic proportions. The cost of Alzheimer's to the US economy is expected to cross a trillion dollars in 10 years. It is a serious health care issue in many of the western countries as the population age and the life expectancy increase.

While this book does not present all the answers, it is an attempt to examines the factors affecting Alzheimer's and how to reduce the risk of developing Alzheimer's. A combination of diet and both mental and physical exercise is believed to help in prevention or reducing risk. The book includes:

Discussion on factors in Alzheimer's development

The list of foods that help protect the brain and boost brain health is included in the book:

Over 30 recipes including teas, smoothies, broths, and other dishes that incorporate brain-boosting foods:

References and links to several research studies on Alzheimer's and brain foods.

ALL NATURAL WELLNESS DRINKS

It contains 35 recipes for wellness drinks that include teas, smoothies, soups, and vegan & bone broths. The recipes in this book are unique and combine superfoods, medicinal spices, and herbs. These drinks are anti-cancer, anti-diabetic, ant-aging, heart healthy, anti-inflammatory, and anti-oxidant as well as promote weight loss.

By infusing nature-based nutrients (super fruits and vegetables, spices, and herbs) into drink recipes, we get some amazing wellness drinks that not only replace water loss but nourish the body with vitamins, essential metals, anti-oxidants, and many other nutrients. These drinks may be further enhanced by incorporating spices and herbs along with other superfoods. These drinks not only help heal the body but also enhance the immune system to help prevent many forms of diseases. These drinks may also help rejuvenate the body and delay the aging process. The book also includes suggested wellness drinks for common ailments.

INTRODUCTION TO CURRY

Curry powder and spice mixes have many health benefits. It has anti-inflammatory, anti-oxidant, anti-cancer and anti-bacterial properties

Curry is becoming a popular dish worldwide. Not only curry is delicious, but it also provides immense health benefits.

Curry powder contains turmeric, chili powder, coriander, and cumin among others. They are all known to have immense health benefits. This book includes:

- History of curry and curry powder
- Health benefits of each ingredient

- How to make various curry powder and curry paste mixes including Indian, Thai, and Ethiopian curry mixes
- Several recipes for making Indian and Thai curries

ESSENTIAL SPICES AND HERBS: GINGER

Ginger is a spice known to man for thousands of years and has been used for cooking and as a natural remedy for common ailments. Recent studies have shown that ginger has anti-cancer, anti-inflammatory, and anti-oxidant properties. Ginger helps in reducing muscle pain and is an excellent remedy for nausea. Ginger promotes a healthy digestive system. The book details:

- Many health benefits of ginger including fighting cancer, inflammation, pain and nausea
- Remedies using ginger
- Recipes for teas, smoothies, and other dishes
- References and links to a number of research studies on the effectiveness of ginger

•

ESSENTIAL SPICES AND HERBS: GARLIC

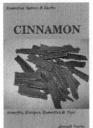 Garlic is one of the worlds healthiest foods. It helps in maintaining a healthy heart, an excellent remedy for common inflections and has both anti-oxidant and anti-inflammatory properties. It is an excellent food supplement that provides some key vitamins and minerals. This book details the benefits of garlic and describes many easy recipes for incorporating garlic into the diet:

- Many health benefits of garlic including fighting cancer, inflammation, heart health and more
- Remedies using garlic
- Recipes for teas, smoothies, and other dishes
- References and links to a number of research studies on the effectiveness of garlic

ESSENTIAL SPICES AND HERBS: CINNAMON

Cinnamon is an essential spice. It has Anti-diabetic, anti-inflammatory, anti-oxidant, anti-cancer and anti-infections and neuroprotective properties. Cinnamon is a spice known to man for thousands of years and has been used for food preservation, baking, cooking, and as a natural remedy for common ailments. Recent studies have shown that cinnamon has important medicinal properties. This book explains:

- Many health benefits of cinnamon including anti-diabetic, neuroprotective and others.
- Recipes for teas, smoothies, and other dishes
- References and links to a number of research studies on the effectiveness of cinnamon

ANTI-CANCER CURRIES

It is estimated that more than 50% of the cancer incidents are preventable by changing lifestyles, controlling or avoiding cancer-causing factors, or simply eating healthy. There are several foods that are known to have anti-cancer properties either directly or indirectly. Some of these have properties that inhibit cancer cell growth while others have anti-oxidant and anti-inflammatory properties that contribute to overall health. However, many spices and herbs have direct anti-cancer properties and when one uses anti-cancer spices and herbs in cooking fresh food, there is an immense benefit to be gained. Curry dishes are cooked using many spices that have anti-oxidant, anti-inflammatory, and anti-cancer properties.

This book contains 30 curry recipes that use healthy and anti-cancer ingredients. These recipes are simple and take an average of 20-30 minutes to prepare.

BEGINNERS GUIDE TO COOKING WITH SPICES

Have you ever wondered how to cook with spices? Learn about the many benefits of spices and how to cook with them!

Find out how to start using spices as seasoning and healthy foods. Includes sample recipes,

Beginner's guide to cooking with spices is an introductory book that explains the history, various uses, and their medicinal properties and health benefits. The book details how they may be easily incorporated in everyday cooking. The book will cover the following:

- Health benefits of spices and herbs
- Spice mixes from around the world and their uses
- Tips for cooking with Spices
- Cooking Vegan with Spices
- Cooking Meat and Fish with spices
- Spiced Rice Dishes
- Spicy Soups and Broths

EASY INDIAN INSTANT POT COOKBOOK

Instant Pot or Electric Pressure Cooker is the most important cooking device in my kitchen. It saves me time, energy, and helps me prepare hassle-free Indian meals all the time.

The Easy Indian Instant Pot Meals contains includes:
- Recipes for 50 Indian dishes
- Tips for cooking with Instant Pot or any electric pressure cooker
- General tips for cooking with spices

FIGHTING THE VIRUS: HOW TO BOOST YOUR BODY'S IMMUNE RESPONSE AND FIGHT VIRUS NATURALLY

What can we do to improve our health and immune response so that our bodies are less prone to viral or bacterial infections? How can we enable our body for a speedy recovery in case of getting such infections?

The answer lies in lifestyle changes that include better hygiene practices, exercise, sleep, and a better diet to keep our body in optimum health. This book is focused on understanding the body's immune system, factors that improve the body's immune response and some natural remedies and recipes. The book contains:
•Overview of the human immune system
•Factors affecting immune response
•Natural substances that fight viral, fungal and bacterial infections
•Recipes that may improve immunity and help speedy recovery
•Supplements that may help improve the immune system
•Scientific studies and references

Easy Spicy Eggs: All Natural Easy and Spicy Egg Recipes

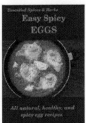Recipes in this book are not a collection of authentic dishes, but a spicy version of chicken recipes that are easy to make and 100% healthy and flavorful. Ingredients used are mostly natural without any preserved or processed foods.

Most of these recipes include tips and tricks to vary and adapt to your taste of spice level or make with some of the ingredients you like other than the prescribed ingredients in the recipes.

There are about 30 recipes in the book with ideas to make another 30 or even more with the suggestions and notes included with many of the recipes. Cooking does not have to be prescriptive but can be creative. I invite you to try your own variations and apply your creativity to cook dishes that are truly your own.

Food for the Brain

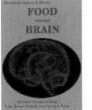Nature provides for foods that nourish both the body and the brain. Most often the focus of the diet is physical

nourishment, - muscle building, weight loss, energy, athletic performance, and many others. Similar to foods that help the body, there are many foods that help the brain, improve memory and help slow down the aging process. While it is normal to have your physical and mental abilities somewhat slow down with age, diseases such as Alzheimer's, and Parkinson's impact these declines even more. Brain function decline accelerates, and more and more brain cells eventually die over time.

With regular exercises, strength training, practicing martial arts and other physical activities can arrest the physical decline. This book's primary focus is on managing decline in mental and brain function through diet and contains the following:
Characteristics of foods that helps in keeping your brain healthy and young. Brain healthy foods including meats, fruits, vegetables, spices, herbs, and seafood. Supplements to improve memory, cognition and support brain health
Mediterranean diet recipe ideas
DASH diet recipe ideas
Asian diet recipe ideas
Brain boosting supplements and recommendations products and dosage
References

Made in the USA
Middletown, DE
03 June 2022